THE ULTIMATE MEAL PREP COOKBOOK FOR WEIGHT LOSS

The Ultimate Beginners Guide to Eating Healthy and Achieving Your Weight Maintenance, which includes a quick, easy diet plan

Adam C.

ISBN: 9798870495392

DEDICATION

This book is dedicated to all my Readers

CONTENTS

Chapter 1: Introduction

1.1 Welcome to the Ultimate Meal Prep Journey

Embark on a life-changing journey to become a healthier and fit version of yourself! Through the power of food preparation, this journey is about embracing a fulfilling and sustainable lifestyle rather than merely losing weight. You'll find the keys to effective weight control, quick and simple meal prep methods, and a ton of delectable recipes catered to your weight loss objectives in the pages that follow.

Meal prep is a deliberate approach to nutrition that gives you the power to take charge of what you eat, not just a fad phrase. Meal planning and preparation in advance takes the guesswork out of eating, lowers the temptation to make bad decisions, and puts you in a successful position to reach and maintain a healthy weight.

Remember that this is a lifestyle change rather than just a temporary solution as we set off on this epic meal prep adventure together. We'll walk you through each step, offering advice, pointers, and selections of recipes that will not only tempt your palate but also help you achieve your weight loss objectives.

1.2 The Importance of Meal Prep for Weight Loss

You may ask, "Why meal prep?" The way it transforms your weight loss journey holds the key to the answer. In a society where convenience foods and rapid living are the norm, meal prep becomes your friend when it comes to attaining sustainable and long-term weight loss. This is why it's so important:

1. Control Your Nutrition: Taking control of your nutrition is possible with meal preparation. You may guarantee a diet rich in nutrients and well-balanced by organizing your meals in advance. Goodbye to careless, unhealthy meal selections and welcome to a thoughtfully planned menu that can help you achieve your weight loss objectives.

2. Easy Portion Control: Portion sizes are frequently one of the main causes of weight gain. Meal planning allows you to precisely measure and manage your servings, which helps you avoid overindulging and stick to your calorie target. It's a straightforward yet powerful tactic that gives you the ability to better control your weight.

3. Efficiency of Time: Meal prep is a time-saving strategy, despite the myth that eating healthily takes more time. Weekly meal prep saves time for other activities and eases the burden of everyday cooking. Set aside a certain block of time for this purpose. It's an investment in your well-being that will pay off in the form of improved wellbeing and time savings.

4. Say Goodbye to Temptation: Imagine having a refrigerator full of wholesome, ready-to-eat meals. This visual feast reduces the temptation to order takeout or grab a quick, less-nutritious snack in addition to making healthy eating more accessible. Preparing your meals helps you create a healthy eating environment that supports your weight loss goals.

5. Financial Savvy: Regular dining out might have a negative financial impact. You may plan meals that are both affordable and nutrient-dense by using meal prep. It's an affordable way to eat healthily that fits with your budget and weight control objectives.

1.3 Setting Your Goals and Expectations

Prior to delving into the realm of food preparation, pause to consider your individual objectives and anticipations. What has led you to this juncture in your path, and what are your goals? Establishing specific objectives helps you stay motivated as you work toward them and gives you a path forward.

1. Define Your Why: Consider your motivation for taking this voyage. Is it to increase your energy, lose extra weight, or enhance your general health? Knowing your "why" will help you stay motivated and customize your meal prep schedule to suit your own requirements.

2. Realistic Expectations: Even if there's a temptation to quick cures, keep in mind that sustained weight loss is a long process. Have reasonable expectations for yourself and concentrate on changing your lifestyle for the better rather than aiming for quick fixes. This method guarantees that you will lose weight and keep it off in the long run.

3. Celebrate Non-Scale Victories: Losing weight is only one part of your journey. Appreciate the little accomplishments along the road, like making a better snack choice, finishing a difficult workout, or adhering to your meal prep schedule. Non-scale wins have a big impact on your success and general well-being.

We'll walk you through the practical side of meal prep in the next chapters, assist you in creating a customized nutrition plan, and provide you a ton of quick and simple recipes. Prepare to enjoy the tastes of a more nutritious way of living as you set out on the best meal prep path for weight loss.

Chapter 2: Understanding the Basics of Weight Loss

2.1 How Weight Loss Works

Knowing the underlying concepts of weight reduction is crucial for anyone starting a weight loss journey that is successful. Understanding how weight reduction works is essential for making informed decisions and achieving long-term success, as it involves a complex interaction of multiple elements.

1. Deficit in Calorie: A calorie deficit is the fundamental idea behind weight reduction. This entails consuming fewer calories than you expend. Your body uses stored energy, mostly fat, to make up for times when it uses more energy than it receives. Effective weight loss starts with creating a calorie deficit, and meal preparation becomes an important tool in reaching this balance.

2. Metabolism and Physical Activity: The process by which your body breaks down food into energy, known as metabolism, is a key component in controlling your weight. Regular exercise increases your metabolism and improves its capacity to burn calories. Including exercise in your regimen improves your general health in addition to helping you lose weight.

3. Hormonal Factors: Hormones control hunger, fullness, and fat storage, among other elements of weight. Gaining knowledge about the effects of hormones like ghrelin, insulin, and leptin on your body might help you develop practical weight-management techniques. Preparing meals with an emphasis on nutrient-dense foods can benefit your weight loss attempts by stabilizing hormone imbalances.

4. Changes to a Sustainable Lifestyle: Although quick fixes like fad diets may seem appealing, long-term lifestyle adjustments are necessary for long-term weight loss. Extreme restriction and crash diets frequently result in short-term success followed by rebound weight gain. Meal prep becomes a game-changer when it comes to developing habits that you can sustain over time.

2.2 The Role of Nutrition in Achieving Weight Goals

The foundation of any effective weight loss plan is nutrition. Your capacity to sustain energy levels, establish a calorie deficit, and promote general well-being is greatly influenced by the foods you eat. Let's examine the essential facets of diet in relation to reaching your weight objectives.

1. Macronutrients: Carbohydrates, Fats, and Proteins: A well-rounded diet must balance the macronutrients proteins, fats, and carbs. Carbohydrates supply quick energy needs, lipids sustain energy levels over time, and proteins aid in the maintenance and repair of muscles. By knowing how to divide these nutrients throughout your meals, you can support weight loss while still meeting your body's needs.

2. Micronutrients: Vitamins and Minerals: Micronutrients, such as vitamins and minerals, are just as important as macronutrients for a variety of physiological processes. A lack of these vital components might impair general health and make weight loss difficult. You can include a variety of fruits, veggies, and whole foods in your meals by prepping them, which will guarantee that you obtain a wide range of micronutrients.

3. Fiber and Satiety: Due to their ability to aid in digestion and promote satiety, foods high in fiber are essential for weight loss. Incorporating high-fiber components into your meal preparation not only prolongs feelings of fullness but also promotes intestinal well-being. Consequently, this enhances the longevity and enjoyment of the process of losing weight.

4. Hydration: It is common to neglect maintaining proper hydration when trying to lose weight. Apart from its physiological benefits, water also has the potential to regulate one's hunger. Our body might occasionally mistake thirst for hunger, which causes us to overindulge in snacks. As you begin your meal planning, don't forget to include adequate water as a cornerstone of your diet.

2.3 Common Myths about Weight Loss and Dieting

There are many myths and misconceptions in the weight loss industry that can lead even the most well-meaning people astray. In order to provide you some clarity and put you on the correct track for long-term weight management, let's dispel a few popular fallacies.

1. Myth: Rapid Weight Loss is Sustainable: Even though losing weight quickly might feel good at first, it's usually not sustainable. Promises of rapid effects from crash diets typically result in muscle loss and a rebound effect when regular eating patterns are resumed. Making long-term lifestyle adjustments is necessary for sustainable weight loss, which is gradual.

2. Myth: Carbohydrates are the Enemy: Reality: Carbohydrates are an essential source of energy, not the enemy. Choosing complex carbs, which are present in whole grains, fruits, and vegetables, helps maintain steady energy levels and delivers vital nutrients. Selecting nutrient-dense foods and exercising moderation are crucial.

3. Myth: Skipping Meals Leads to Weight Loss: The truth is that missing meals can mess with your metabolism, which might cause you to overeat later in the day. Preparing meals in advance promotes consistent, well-balanced eating, suppresses excessive hunger, and speeds up metabolism. Maintaining a regular eating schedule is essential for effective weight loss.

4. Myth: All Calories are Created Equal: Reality: Although a caloric deficit is a basic idea, the type of calorie counts. Foods high in nutrients not only help you meet your calorie targets but also supply vital vitamins and minerals. Paying attention to the nutritional content of your meals improves your weight reduction plan's overall efficacy.

5. Myth: Exercise Alone Guarantees Weight Loss: Reality: While exercise is an essential part of a healthy lifestyle, it cannot be used as a stand-alone weight loss strategy. The best outcomes are obtained when a balanced diet and frequent exercise are combined. By ensuring that your nutrition supports your fitness activities, meal prep helps to support this synergy.

We'll go into more detail on how to apply these ideas to your meal planning routine in the upcoming chapters. Knowing the fundamentals of weight loss gives you the power to make wise decisions, laying the groundwork for an effective and long-lasting road to a healthy you.

Chapter 3: Getting Started with Healthy Eating

Well done for starting down the path to a better living! This chapter will cover the fundamentals of healthy eating, giving you the information and resources you need to create a plate that is balanced, comprehend the nutrients you need to lose weight, and put sensible portion management techniques into practice.

3.1 Building a Balanced Plate

The foundation of a healthy diet is assembling a plate that is balanced. It supports your weight loss objectives while making sure you obtain a variety of nutrients required for general well-being. It's important to include a variety of macro and micronutrients in each meal. Let's dissect what makes a plate balanced:

1. Fill Half Your Plate with Vegetables: Because they are high in fiber, vitamins, and minerals, vegetables are an essential part of a diet that is balanced. You can eat a satisfying number of them without going overboard because they are high in volume and low in calories. To guarantee a wide range of nutrients, try to incorporate a colorful assortment of veggies.

2. Include Lean Proteins: For the upkeep, repair, and satisfaction of muscles, proteins are necessary. Include lean protein sources in your diet, such as beans, low-fat dairy, fish, poultry, and tofu. Additionally, protein has a stronger thermic impact than other foods, which means that digesting it takes more energy and adds to the process of burning calories.

3. Choose Whole Grains: Complex carbs, fiber, and vital minerals are all found in whole grains. Refined grains should be avoided in favor of whole grains such as brown rice, quinoa, oats, and whole wheat bread. These options help you maintain your energy levels and prevent overeating by extending your feeling of fullness.

4. Add Healthy Fats: It's important to watch portion sizes, but it's also important to include healthy fats in your diet. Good sources of mono- and polyunsaturated fats include avocados, almonds, seeds, and olive oil. These fats promote general health, cognitive function, and food absorption.

5. Don't Forget About Dairy or Dairy Alternatives: For healthy bones, dairy products and their fortified counterparts are a good source of calcium and vitamin D. Select options that are low in fat or fat free to control your calorie consumption and yet get the benefits of these vital nutrients.

6. Be Mindful of Portion Sizes: Portion control is essential for controlling calorie consumption even while creating a balanced plate. Thoughtfully calculating portion sizes guarantees that you get the proper quantity of nutrients without going overboard. We'll go into more detail about portion control techniques in the following section.

7. Hydration Matters: Drinking enough water is an essential component of eating a nutritious diet, even if it's not on the plate. Water promotes general health, aids in hunger control, and aids in digestion. Limit the amount of sugar-filled beverages you consume and make water your main beverage option.

When preparing meals, concentrate on making dishes that are aesthetically pleasing, full of different nutrients, and pleasing to the palate. Try a variety of food pairings to add interest and enjoyment to your meals.

3.2 Essential Nutrients for Weight Loss

Knowing how important nutrients are to losing weight gives you the ability to plan meals with knowledge and confidence. Let's examine some essential nutrients that are critical to achieving your weight loss objectives:

1. Protein: One of the best nutrients for losing weight is protein. It is essential for maintaining lean muscle mass and helps you feel fuller for extended periods of time by promoting satiety. Incorporate foods high in protein into every meal to aid in your weight loss efforts.

2. Fiber: Your ally in managing your weight is fiber. It gives your diet more substance, which encourages satiety and keeps you from overeating. In addition, fiber promotes healthy digestion and blood sugar regulation. Legumes, fruits, vegetables, and whole grains are all great sources of dietary fiber.

3. Healthy Fats: Healthy fats are crucial for both weight loss and general health, despite the common belief that all fats are bad. They aid in the creation of hormones, promote nutritional absorption, and aid in satiety. Incorporate healthy fat sources into your meals, such as nuts, avocados, and olive oil.

4. Vitamins and Minerals: A wide variety of vitamins and minerals are essential for many physiological processes, such as energy production and metabolism. Consuming an array of fruits, vegetables, lean meats, and whole grains guarantees that your body gets a wide range of these vital elements.

5. Water: Water is essential for weight loss even though it isn't a nutrient in the conventional sense. Maintaining proper hydration promotes a healthy metabolism, regulates hunger, and keeps your body operating at its best. Make it a point to stay hydrated during the day, especially in the hours before meals.

6. Calcium and Vitamin D: For strong bones, calcium and vitamin D are important, and when losing weight, their importance increases. To make sure you're getting enough of these nutrients, including dairy or fortified substitutes in your diet.

3.3 Portion Control Strategies

A key component of successful weight management is portion control. It keeps you inside your calorie target range and stops you from overeating. The following useful tips can help you incorporate portion control into your meals:

1. Use Smaller Plates: How much you eat might be affected by the size of your plate. Employing smaller dishes creates the appearance of a larger plate, encouraging contentment with reduced serving sizes.

2. Measure Portions: Purchasing a kitchen scale and measuring cups can be helpful resources for managing serving quantities. Even while you don't have to measure every bite, using it occasionally helps you understand the right portion proportions.

3. Follow the Plate Method: Make portions on your plate for each food group. As an illustration, divide the plate in half for veggies, quarters for lean protein, and quarters for whole grains. This technique encourages balance by using visual cues to guide portion amounts.

4. Be Mindful of Liquid Calories: Alcohol and sugar-filled drinks are two examples of liquid calories that can make a big difference in your daily intake. Take note of these sources and think about choosing low-calorie drinks like water or herbal tea.

5. Listen to Your Body: Observe your body's signals of hunger and fullness. Savor each bite as you eat gently, and stop when you're full. This mindful eating strategy aids in reducing overindulgence.

6. Pre-portion Snacks: Make sure to portion your snacks into individual servings while preparing them for the week. This method gives precise instructions on serving amounts and removes the temptation to eat straight out of the bag.

7. Plan Balanced Snacks: To improve fullness, incorporate a balance of macronutrients in your snacks. For instance, have yogurt with a dusting of oats or a tiny quantity of nuts and fruit.

As you implement these portion control techniques, keep in mind that harmony is essential. The objective is to assist your weight loss journey and foster a positive relationship with food, not to deprive you.

We'll delve more into the how-to of meal prep in the following chapters, assisting you in putting these ideas into practice to make scrumptious and nourishing meals that support your weight loss objectives. Remember that every thoughtful portion and well-balanced plate you put in puts you one step closer to reaching and maintaining your target weight as you move forward with your healthy lifestyle path.

Chapter4: The Ultimate Meal Prep Guide

This is where your adventure really begins the comprehensive approach to meal prep for weight loss. This chapter will walk you through the process of organizing your weekly meals, highlight the many advantages meal prep offers for your weight reduction endeavors, and offer helpful advice on how to make your meal prep sessions run smoothly.

4.1 Benefits of Meal Prep for Weight Loss

Meal prep is not only a time-saving method; it's a potent tactic that can greatly influence your capacity to lose weight and keep it off. Let's examine the many advantages that make meal preparation a game-changer on your path to better health:

1. Portion Control Made Simple: Regulation of portion sizes is one of the problems associated with weight management. Meal prep eliminates uncertainty by preparing your meals and snacks in advance. By doing this, you can be sure that you're getting the proper quantity of calories and nutrients to support your weight loss efforts.

2. Nutrient-Dense Choices: Making meals ahead of time allows you to choose foods that are nutrient-dense and thoughtful. Lean proteins, whole grains, healthy fats, and a range of vibrant veggies may all be included in your meals to create a well-balanced diet that will help you lose weight.

3. Reduced Temptation for Unhealthy Options: Having pre-made meals available lessens the temptation to choose less healthful options in a society where food fast and easy-to-make but frequently harmful options abound.

4. Time-Saving Convenience: It can be difficult to find time in a busy life to prepare nutritious meals every day. Meal prep simplifies the process and lets you set aside a certain time each week to make meals. This convenient way to save time helps you achieve your weight loss objectives and free up time for other important things.

5. Consistency in Nutrition: To lose weight, consistency is essential. Meal preparation guarantees that you provide your body the correct nutrients in the proper amounts on a regular basis. This regularity speeds up your metabolism, controls hunger, and helps you maintain your weight over the long run.

6. Financial Benefits: Regularly dining out or getting takeaway might be expensive. Meal prep is a cheap fix that helps you buy items in bulk, plan your meals, and reduce food waste. As a result, you make deliberate decisions about the quality of your ingredients in addition to saving money.

7. Customization for Dietary Goals: Meal prep enables customization, regardless of whether you're adhering to a certain diet or have particular nutritional demands. It is simpler to follow your nutritional objectives when you are in charge of the components, serving sizes, and general arrangement of your meals.

4.2 Planning Your Weekly Meals

Meal prep that works starts with careful planning, weekly meal planning guarantees that your menu is well-balanced and satisfying, and it also sets the stage for success. Here's a detailed guide to assist you in organizing your weekly meal plan:

1. Assess Your Schedule: Begin by thinking about the upcoming week. Make a note of the days you may or may not have more time to prepare meals. Determine any obstacles or occasions that can make it difficult for you to follow your eating plan.

2. Set Realistic Goals: Regarding the amount of time and effort you can devote to meal prep, be reasonable. Long-term maintenance of your meal prep habit is ensured by setting realistic goals. If you've never prepared meals before, start small and work your way up to preparing more meals each week as you get more accustomed to it.

3. Choose Balanced Recipes: Choose dishes that include a range of food groups, such as whole grains, lean proteins, vegetables, and healthy fats. In addition to helping you achieve your weight loss objectives and offering a varied and pleasurable dining experience, this guarantees that your meals are nutritionally balanced.

4. Create a Shopping List: Make a grocery list based on the ingredients required for the recipes you've selected. Sort the list into sections like grains, fruits, proteins, and pantry staples. By using a methodical approach, you may shop for groceries more efficiently and are less likely to forget important products.

5. Prep for Success: Make sure your preparation schedule takes into account the particular requirements of the recipes you have selected. Certain components can be marinated, chopped, or cooked partially ahead of time. This preparation guarantees a more seamless cooking procedure and saves time throughout the workweek.

6. Embrace Variety: Not only is variety the flavor of life, but it's also essential to eating a balanced diet. To avoid boredom and keep your palate interested, schedule a variety of meals throughout the week that feature different tastes, textures, and cuisines.

7. Factor in Leftovers: Make bigger batches of some dishes with the intention of using the leftovers for lunch or dinner the following day. This tactic lowers the need to cook every day while increasing efficiency.

8. Stay Flexible: Though planning is necessary, things happen in life. Be adaptable and willing to make changes. Adjust your strategy in case of unforeseen circumstances or if you have leftovers from a prior supper.

4.3 Tips for Efficient and Effective Meal Prep

Making meal preps a fun and sustainable part of your routine requires efficiency. You may optimize the efficiency of your meal prep sessions by following these tips:

1. Invest in Quality Containers: You can properly portion and store your meals if you have a range of containers in various sizes. For added convenience, choose microwave and dishwasher safe containers.

2. Batch Cooking: Cooking in batches entails making several portions of a dish at once. By using this method, you may stock your freezer or fridge with meals that are ready to eat for the upcoming week while also saving time.

3. Use Time-Saving Kitchen Tools: Invest in kitchen appliances that will save you time, such a food processor, a vegetable peeler, and a decent knife. Meal prep may be done much more quickly and efficiently with the help of this equipment.

4. Cook in Stages: Preparing meals doesn't have to take all day. Divide it into phases that are doable. You could, for instance, chop veggies one day, marinate proteins the next, and then put meals together the following day.

5. Embrace One-Pan and One-Pot Recipes: Select recipes that can be prepared in a single skillet or pot to streamline your dinner prep. This expedites the cooking process and reduces clean up as well.

6. Plan for Theme Nights: Set aside particular nights for themes, such "Mexican Monday" or "Stir-Fry Friday." This method simplifies meal planning and increases meal diversity.

7. Utilize Your Freezer: Not every meal must be finished in a few days. A lot of dishes freeze nicely, so you can prepare ahead of time meals for busy days.

8. Make it a Social Activity: Ask loved ones to assist you with food preparation. By sharing the workload, you can turn it into a fun and social activity that also improves process efficiency.

9. Plan for Flexibility: Even while structure is crucial, allow for some flexibility. You can modify your plan to suit your tastes if you're not in the mood for a particular meal by having substitute options or ingredients.

As you begin your meal preparation adventure, keep in mind that perfection comes from practice. It's common to have difficulties at first, but with practice and time, you'll create a schedule that works for your tastes and way of life. Meal prep has advantages that go beyond only helping people lose weight; they also cover a wide range of health and wellbeing topics. You'll find a variety of quick and simple recipes in the next chapters that will help you achieve your weight loss objectives and improve your meal prep experience. Prepare to enjoy the tastes of a more nutritious way of living!

Chapter 5: Creating Your Quick and Easy Diet Plan

We'll explore the fascinating world of creating a customized nutrition plan that supports your weight loss objectives in this chapter. We'll discuss how variation contributes to nutrient diversity and present you a selection of quick and simple meals that are perfect for hectic schedules.

5.1 Designing a Personalized Diet Plan

Creating a customized nutrition plan is a crucial step in achieving long-term weight loss. Although there isn't a single strategy that works for everyone, you can follow these guidelines to help you create a plan that suits your tastes, way of life, and health requirements:

1. Assess Your Dietary Preferences and Restrictions: Think about your nutritional choices, including the items you like and would like to eat more of in your meals. Make a note of any dietary limitations or medical issues that might affect the foods you choose. A diet that suits your preferences and works with any limitations is more likely to last.

2. Determine Your Caloric Needs: Knowing how many calories you need each day is essential for managing your weight. You need to consider factors like age, gender, exercise level, and weight loss objectives when calculating how many calories you need. You can estimate your daily caloric needs by using online calculators or by speaking with a nutritionist. This will provide you a starting point for creating your diet plan.

3. Set Macronutrient Ratios: Although there isn't a precise macronutrient ratio that works for everyone, you can establish general parameters based on your lifestyle and tastes. It is common for a balanced macronutrient distribution to contain moderate levels of healthy fats, carbs, and proteins. Try out several ratios to see what suits you the best.

4. Plan Your Meals and Snacks: Your daily calorie intake should be split between meals and snacks. Not only can meal planning help you consume fewer calories overall, but it also guarantees a steady supply of nutrients throughout the day. Every meal should contain a variety of entire grains, fruits, vegetables, lean meats, and healthy fats.

5. Be Mindful of Portion Sizes: Portion control is still essential, even with a well-thought-out diet plan. Pay attention to portion proportions to prevent overindulging. To keep portion constancy, think about utilizing instruments like measuring cups or visual clues (such estimating protein doses with your hand).

6. Hydration: Remember how important it is to stay hydrated. In addition to being good for general health, water can also make you feel full. Make water your main beverage of choice and take into account how hydrated items like fruits and veggies are.

7. Gradual Changes: To prevent feeling overwhelmed when switching from a different eating pattern, think about making little adjustments at first. As your palate and habits change over time, begin by introducing one or two new habits each week.

8. Listen to Your Body: Observe your body's signals of hunger and fullness. Consume food only when you're hungry and quit when you're full. This mindful eating strategy encourages a positive connection with food and honors your body's natural cues.

5.2 Incorporating Variety for Nutrient Diversity

In addition to being a necessary component of a fulfilling and nutritionally varied diet, variety is known as the spice of life. Including a range of foods in your meals guarantees that you get a wide range of nutrients, which improves your general health and wellbeing, here's how to add some diversity to your diet:

1. Explore Different Food Groups: Incorporate a variety of food categories into your diet. Accept a diet rich in color-dense fruits and vegetables, lean meats and seafood, whole grains like quinoa and brown rice, and healthy fats from nuts and avocados.

2. Seasonal Eating: Benefit from stuff that is in season. In addition to having the best flavor, seasonal fruits and vegetables are also packed with nutrients. Go to your neighborhood farmers' markets to find in-season, fresh produce.

3. Try New Recipes and Cuisines: Try out various dishes and learn about international cuisines. Attempting new recipes not only livens up your meals but also broadens your diet by introducing a range of flavors and ingredients.

4. Mix up Cooking Methods: Change up your cooking techniques to bring out the flavors and textures of your food. Try steaming for a light and fresh meal, grilling proteins for a smokey flavor, or roasting veggies for a caramelized sweetness.

5. Rainbow on Your Plate: Try to make a platter that is vibrant. The presence of different antioxidants and phytonutrients is indicated by the colors of fruits and vegetables. Your dish will look more colorful and your intake of nutrients will be more varied.

6. Alternate Protein Sources: Although lean meats are an excellent source of protein, you should also think about including other protein sources like lentils, tofu, and tempeh. These choices offer a range of textures and flavors in addition to varying your nutrient intake.

7. Whole, Unprocessed Foods: Pick complete, unprocessed foods whenever you can. These foods help to create a diet that is both nutrient-dense and well-rounded since they hold onto their original flavors and nutrients.

8. Weekly Rotation: Establish a weekly food plan with a variety of grains, veggies, and proteins. This rotation streamlines your meal planning process and guarantees diversity.

5.3 Quick and Easy Recipes for Busy Lifestyles

In a world when people have hectic schedules, quick and simple dishes are crucial to eating a balanced diet. The main goals of these recipes are to be tasty, time-saving, and convenient. Here are some quick and simple dishes to add to your weekly meal prep routine:

1. Sheet Pan Chicken and Vegetables

Ingredients:

- Chicken breasts or thighs
- Assorted vegetables (bell peppers, broccoli, cherry tomatoes)
- Olive oil
- Garlic powder, paprika, salt, and pepper for seasoning

Instructions:

1. Preheat the oven to 400°F (200°C).

2. Place chicken and chopped vegetables on a sheet pan.

3. Drizzle with olive oil and sprinkle with garlic powder, paprika, salt, and pepper.

4. Toss everything together to ensure even coating.

5. Bake for 20-25 minutes or until the chicken is cooked through and vegetables are tender.

2. Quinoa Salad with Chickpeas and Mediterranean Flavors

Ingredients:

- Cooked quinoa
- Canned chickpeas, drained and rinsed
- Cherry tomatoes, halved
- Cucumber, diced
- Red onion, finely chopped
- Kalamata olives, sliced
- Feta cheese, crumbled
- Olive oil, lemon juice, salt, and pepper for dressing

Instructions:

1. In a large bowl, combine cooked quinoa, chickpeas, tomatoes, cucumber, red onion, olives, and feta.

2. In a small bowl, whisk together olive oil, lemon juice, salt, and pepper for the dressing.

3. Pour the dressing over the salad and toss to combine.

3. Stir-Fry with Tofu and Mixed Vegetables

Ingredients:

- Firm tofu, cubed
- Mixed stir-fry vegetables (bell peppers, broccoli, snap peas, carrots)
- Soy sauce, sesame oil, and ginger for seasoning
- Cooked brown rice or quinoa

Instructions:

1. Press tofu to remove excess water, and then cube it.
2. Stir-fry tofu in a pan until golden brown.
3. Add mixed vegetables to the pan and continue to stir-fry until tender-crisp.
4. Season with soy sauce and a splash of sesame oil. Add grated ginger for flavor.
5. Serve over cooked brown rice or quinoa.

4. Spinach and Feta Stuffed Chicken Breast

Ingredients:

- Chicken breasts
- Fresh spinach leaves
- Feta cheese, crumbled

- Garlic powder, oregano, salt, and pepper for seasoning

Instructions:

1. Preheat the oven to 375°F (190°C).
2. Butterfly the chicken breasts.
3. Layer fresh spinach and crumbled feta on one half of each chicken breast.
4. Fold the other half over the filling and secure with toothpicks.
5. Season the outside of the chicken with garlic powder, oregano, salt, and pepper.
6. Bake for 25-30 minutes or until the chicken is cooked through.

5. Shrimp and Vegetable Skewers

Ingredients:

- Shrimp, peeled and deveined
- Bell peppers, cherry tomatoes, zucchini, and red onion, cut into chunks
- Olive oil, lemon juice, garlic, salt, and pepper for marinade

Instructions:

1. In a bowl, combine shrimp and chopped vegetables.

2. In a separate bowl, whisk together olive oil, lemon juice, minced garlic, salt, and pepper.

3. Pour the marinade over the shrimp and vegetables. Toss to coat evenly.

4. Thread shrimp and vegetables onto skewers.

5. Grill or bake for 8-10 minutes, turning halfway through.

6. Overnight Oats with Berries and Almonds

Ingredients:

- Old-fashioned oats
- Greek yogurt
- Milk (dairy or plant-based)
- Honey or maple syrup
- Mixed berries (strawberries, blueberries, raspberries)
- Sliced almonds

Instructions:

- In a jar or container, combine oats, Greek yogurt, milk, and a drizzle of honey or maple syrup. Mix well.
- Add mixed berries and sliced almonds on top.
- Cover and refrigerate overnight.
- Enjoy a quick and nutritious breakfast the next morning.

These are merely suggestions at this moment. You are welcome to alter them to suit your dietary needs and tastes. The secret is to make sure your meals are tasty, straightforward, and in line with your weight loss objectives.

Stay flexible as you incorporate these simple and quick meals into your customized nutrition plan. Make the recipes your own, play around with the ingredients, and savor the process of trying out new flavors. Making the switch to a healthier lifestyle should be fulfilling, pleasurable, and long-lasting. We'll continue to look at delectable recipes and useful advice to improve your meal planning experience in the upcoming chapters. Prepare to enjoy the benefits of a healthy, well-balanced diet!

Chapter 6: Meal Prep Tools and Techniques

In addition to wholesome meals and careful preparation, effective meal prep also requires the appropriate equipment and methods to speed up the process. This chapter will go over the necessary kitchen gear for meal preparation, time-saving practices to get the most out of your work, and batch cooking and freezing procedures to make sure you always have wholesome options available.

6.1 Essential Kitchen Tools for Meal Prep

Meal prep sessions can be much more efficient if you have the proper tools in your kitchen. The following is a list of necessary appliances for a well-stocked meal prep kitchen:

1. Quality Knives: Invest in a good quality knife set that comes with a serrated knife, paring knife, and chef's knife. You can save time and work by using sharp knives to chop and slice food more precisely and efficiently.

2. Cutting Boards: Cross-contamination can be avoided by keeping different kinds of ingredients apart with a variety of cutting boards. Select reusable, stain-resistant cutting boards in a range of sizes.

3. Measuring Cups and Spoons: To regulate portions and make sure your recipes turn out the way you intended, precise measures are essential measurement cups and spoons are essential tools for anyone who enjoys food prep.

4. Food Storage Containers: Invest in a range of sealed, high-quality food storage containers in different sizes. To maintain the freshness and organization of your prepared meals and components, these containers are crucial for portioning and storing them.

5. Sheet Pans and Baking Trays: When it comes to roasting veggies, baking proteins, and making one-pan meals, sheet pans and baking trays come in handy. For simple clean up, choose lined or non-stick alternatives.

6. Mixing Bowls: Tossing salads, marinating proteins, and mixing ingredients all require a variety of sizes of mixing bowls. Select bowls that are robust and simple to maintain.

7. Kitchen Scale: For accurate measurements, a kitchen scale is an invaluable tool, particularly for portion management. It guarantees uniformity in your recipes and assists you in measuring components precisely.

8. Blender or Food Processor: A food processor or blender is an incredibly useful appliance for making purees, sauces, dressings, and smoothies. It can speed up some activities and reduce the amount of time spent chopping.

9. Slow Cooker or Instant Pot: When it comes to meal planning, a slow cooker or Instant Pot might be your saving grace. They let you whip up big pots of soups, stews, and other recipes quickly and with little effort.

10. Mandoline Slicer: A mandoline slicer is a useful instrument for slicing vegetables evenly and rapidly. When you need thin, uniform slices for salads or other foods, it's really helpful.

11. Herb and Spice Containers: Seasoning food is made easy when you have an orderly spice and herb cabinet. To make it simple to locate and recognize your preferred tastes, use clear containers.

12. Vegetable Peeler: To peel and prepare a wide variety of vegetables fast and effectively, you'll need a decent vegetable peeler.

13. Citrus Juicer: A citrus juicer can make it easy and efficient to extract juice for recipes that call for fresh citrus without the trouble of hand-squeezing the juice.

14. Kitchen Timer: A kitchen timer may help you stay on track during meal prep, ensuring that each component is cooked or prepped for the proper length of time.

15. Thermometer: A kitchen thermometer is vital for testing the internal temperature of proteins to ensure they are cooked safely and to perfection.

Having these important items in your kitchen armory sets you up for success in your food prep attempts. Consider the individual needs of your recipes and tastes when selecting additional instruments to tailor your kitchen setup.

6.2 Time-Saving Meal Prep Techniques

Time is sometimes a limiting factor when it comes to cooking meals, but with clever tactics, you may make the most of the time you have. Here are time-saving meal prep ideas to include into your routine:

1. Prep and Chop in Batches: Rather than cutting ingredients for each dish separately, group your prep work. For example, cut all your vegetables at once and keep them in separate containers until you're ready to use them. This saves time on clean up and repetitive duties.

2. Use Frozen Vegetables: While fresh vegetables are excellent, frozen vegetables are a simple and time-saving option. They are pre-washed and pre-chopped, avoiding the need for substantial prep work. Simply thaw or cook them immediately from frozen.

3. Pre-marinate Proteins: Marinating proteins in advance not only increases flavor but also saves time on the day of preparation. Place meats like chicken, fish, or tofu in marinades and store them in the fridge until you're ready to cook.

4. One-Pan and One-Pot Meals: Opt for meals that can be cooked in a single pan or pot. These meals not only save time on preparing but also limit the amount of dishes to clean. Sheet pan dinners, stir-fries, and casseroles are wonderful possibilities.

5. Pre-portion Snacks: When making snacks for the week, separate them into individual containers or snack-sized bags. This eliminates the need to measure each time you grab a snack and improves portion control.

6. Cook Once, Eat Twice: Embrace the concept of cooking once and eating twice. Prepare larger batches of recipes and use leftovers for following dinners. For example, roast additional veggies to add to salads or use cooked quinoa in different meals throughout the week.

7. Utilize Pre-cooked Ingredients: Incorporate pre-cooked products like rotisserie chicken, canned beans, or pre-cooked grains into your dishes. These items greatly cut down on cooking time and are convenient complements to diverse recipes.

8. Time-Saving Kitchen Gadgets: Explore time-saving kitchen tools like a garlic press, vegetable chopper, or egg slicer. While not essential, these tools can speed up key activities, making meal prep more efficient.

9. Plan for Multitasking: Maximize your time in the kitchen by multitasking. While one component is cooking, utilize that opportunity to chop veggies, measure ingredients, or clean up. Efficient utilization of time can make the overall process smoother.

10. Create a Weekly Routine: Establish a weekly plan for meal prep to generate a sense of structure. Designate distinct days for planning, shopping, and prepping. Consistency in your routine helps streamline the process over time.

6.3 Batch Cooking and Freezing Strategies

Batch cooking and freezing are excellent tactics for ensuring that you always have nutritious and ready-to-eat meals at your disposal. Here's how to efficiently include batch cooking and freezing into your meal planning routine:

1. Batch Cooking Basics: Batch cooking includes creating bigger quantities of recipes than you need for a single meal. This strategy allows you to save additional servings for future use. Choose recipes that freeze well and can be readily reheated without compromising quality.

2. Meal Prep Sessions: Set aside specific meal planning sessions during the week to focus on batch cooking. Use these sessions to cook proteins, cereals, and other components in quantity. This not only saves time but also provides a consistent supply of pre-cooked ingredients.

3. Portion and Label: After batch cooking, separate your dishes into individual servings. Use airtight containers or freezer bags to keep freshness. Label each container with the date and contents to easily identify what's inside.

4. Freeze Flat: When freezing liquids or soups, freeze them flat in freezer bags. This strategy provides for quicker thawing and saves room in the freezer. Once frozen, the bags can be stacked vertically.

5. Use Freezer-Friendly Containers: Invest in freezer-friendly containers that can resist freezing temperatures without shattering. Glass containers with lockable closures or high-quality plastic containers are great for freezing meals.

6. Flash Freezing: For goods that are individually portioned, consider flash freezing. Place items like berries or individual proteins on a tray and freeze them until solid before transferring to a freezer bag. This stops objects from staying together.

7. Keep an Inventory: Maintain a freezer inventory to track the contents of your freezer. This helps you keep track of what you have on hand and prevents goods from being forgotten or neglected.

8. Thawing Strategies: Plan your meals in advance and thaw frozen foods in the refrigerator overnight. Alternatively, utilize the defrost option on your microwave for rapid thawing. Avoid thawing at room temperature to guarantee food safety.

9. Label with Expiry Dates: Label frozen foods with expiry dates to maintain quality. While frozen meals can last for an extended period, labeling ensures that you prioritize consuming older foods first.

10. Variety in Freezer Stock: Create a broad range of frozen meals to cater to different interests and moods having a variety of options guarantees that you always have a nice and savory supper ready.

11. Reheat with Care: When reheating frozen meals, do so with care to maintain texture and flavor. Use the proper method microwave, oven, or stovetop—and follow specified parameters for each dish.

Batch cooking and freezing not only save time but also provide a safety net for hectic days when preparing from scratch is tough. With these tactics, you can develop a freezer stocked with nutritious, handmade meals that correspond with your weight loss objectives.

As you integrate these meal prep tools and practices into your routine, remember that the key to successful meal prep is consistency and adaptation. Tailor these tactics to fit your lifestyle, experiment with new tools, and embrace the process of discovering what works best for you. In the future chapters, we'll continue to explore great recipes and other techniques to enrich your meal planning adventure. Get ready to enjoy the benefits of a well-organized and effective meal planning routine!

Chapter 7: Overcoming Common Challenges

Embarking on a road toward weight loss and healthy eating through meal prep is a praiseworthy attempt, but it comes with its share of hurdles. In this chapter, we'll examine major difficulties that many persons confront and suggest practical solutions to overcome them. From controlling cravings and emotional eating to staying motivated and navigating social situations, you'll acquire insights to make your path more robust and fun.

7.1 Dealing with Cravings and Emotional Eating

Cravings and emotional eating can pose substantial hurdles to keeping a balanced diet. Understanding the core causes and implementing mindful solutions will help you traverse these difficulties efficiently.

1. Recognizing Cravings vs. Hunger: Distinguishing between actual hunger and cravings is the first step in tackling this difficulty. Hunger is a physiological need for sustenance, but cravings are often induced by psychological or emotional factors. Before grabbing for a snack, ask yourself if you're actually hungry or if there's an emotional component driving the impulse to eat.

2. Mindful Eating Practices: Practicing mindful eating can help you become more receptive to your body's messages. Take the time to taste each bite, chew gently, and pay attention to the flavors and textures of your food. Mindful eating fosters a deeper connection with your food and can lessen the risk of succumbing to impulsive cravings.

3. Addressing Emotional Triggers: Emotional eating is a frequent response to stress, boredom, melancholy, or other emotions. Identify your emotional triggers and explore alternate strategies to cope with them. Engaging in activities like meditation, fitness, or creative hobbies might give better channels for emotional expression.

4. Having Healthy Alternatives: When cravings arise, having healthy options on hand can be a game-changer. Stock your kitchen with nutrient-dense snacks like fresh fruit, raw almonds, or Greek yogurt. These solutions can satisfy cravings while adding to your overall dietary objectives.

5. Moderation, Not Deprivation: Depriving yourself of certain foods might exacerbate desires. Instead of rigorous deprivation, practice moderation. Allow yourself to enjoy tiny servings of your favorite foods sometimes, relishing the experience without compromising your overall nutritional goals.

6. Stay Hydrated: Thirst can sometimes be confused for hunger or urges. Ensure you stay appropriately hydrated throughout the day. Drinking water can help suppress misleading hunger signals and add to your general well-being.

7. Seek Support: If emotional eating becomes a persistent concern, consider seeking support from friends, family, or a mental health professional. Having a support system can provide encouragement, accountability, and direction in managing emotional elements of your relationship with food.

7.2 Staying Motivated on Your Weight Loss Journey

Sustaining motivation during your weight loss journey is vital for long-term success. Here are techniques to help you keep motivated and focused on your goals.

1. Define Clear Goals: Clearly identify your weight loss and health goals. Whether it's hitting a certain weight, boosting exercise levels, or creating healthy eating habits, having defined and quantifiable goals gives a blueprint for your path.

2. Celebrate Small Wins: Acknowledge and celebrate your victories along the road. Whether it's completing a fitness milestone, regularly following to your meal prep routine, or making healthier food choices, recognizing and celebrating minor triumphs supports your progress.

3. Create a Supportive Environment: Surround yourself with a supportive environment that coincides with your aims. Share your ambitions with friends and family who can provide encouragement and understanding. Consider joining a fitness group or online community to interact with like-minded individuals.

4. Establish Routine and Habits: Incorporate healthful behaviors into your regular routine. Establishing a consistent food prep plan, committing time for physical activity, and prioritizing self-care become engrained habits that add to your overall well-being.

5. Track Your Progress: Documenting your progress, whether through a journal, photos, or tracking applications, encourage you to visualize the good improvements occurring. Reflecting on how far you've gone can be a tremendous motivator during hard times.

6. Set Realistic Expectations: Set realistic and achievable expectations for your weight loss journey. Rapid, abrupt changes can be difficult to sustain and may lead to frustration. Focus on slow, sustained improvement that matches with your own speed and preferences.

7. Mix up Your Routine: Combat monotony by introducing variation into your routine. Explore new cuisines, try different forms of exercise, or set new tasks for yourself. Keeping your routine varied and entertaining minimizes boredom and promotes motivation.

8. Visualize Your Success: Create a mental vision of your success. Visualization may be a strong tool in reaffirming your commitment to your goals. Envision yourself completing milestones, feeling well, and enjoying the pleasant effects of your work.

9. Adjust Goals as Needed: Flexibility is crucial in a weight loss program. Life conditions, priorities, and preferences may vary over time. Be open to altering your goals to correspond with your evolving needs while retaining an emphasis on overall well-being.

7.3 Handling Social Situations and Dining Out

Navigating social situations and dining out can provide hurdles when seeking to maintain a healthy eating pattern. These ideas will help you make attentive choices without feeling confined.

1. Plan Ahead: Before attending social events or dining out, plan ahead by examining menus or inquiring about the available options. This allows you to make informed choices that match with your nutritional goals.

2. Choose Wisely: Opt for nutrient-dense choices whenever possible. Look for dishes that include lean proteins, vegetables, and nutritious grains. Many restaurants provide healthier choices or adaptations to fit dietary requirements.

3. Control Portion Sizes: Restaurants often serve greater servings than necessary. Be aware of portion sizes and consider sharing dishes or asking for a to-go box to store up leftovers before starting your dinner.

4. Listen to Your Hunger Cues: Pay attention to your body's hunger cues and eat mindfully. Pause between mouthful, relish the tastes, and recognize when you're comfortably content. This approach helps reduce overeating in social circumstances.

5. Communicate Your Goals: Share your health and fitness objectives with friends and family. Communicating your aims creates understanding and may motivate others to make healthy choices as well.

6. Bring a Dish: When attending events, offer to provide a dish. This guarantees that you have a healthy option available and helps you to participate to the event in a positive way.

7. Limit Alcohol Intake: Alcoholic beverages can contribute considerable calories to your overall intake. Consume alcohol in moderation and consider alternating with water or other non-caloric beverages.

8. Be Mindful of Treats: It's great to enjoy treats in social circumstances, but be cautious of your selections. Opt for smaller servings or split desserts to satiate your sweet desire without derailing your efforts.

9. Stay Active: Incorporate physical activities into social events wherever possible. Whether it's a post-meal walk or participating in group activities, staying active contributes to your general well-being.

10. Practice Flexibility: Maintain a flexible mindset when presented with unexpected dining circumstances or social occasions. It's normal to depart from your schedule occasionally, as long as you return to your good behaviors afterward.

11. Enjoy the Experience: Focus on the social aspects of gatherings and dining out. Enjoy the company of people, participate in meaningful conversations, and relish the event rather than fixating simply on the food.

By proactively tackling these typical problems, you'll build resilience and adaptability on your journey to weight loss and healthy living. Remember that progress is a dynamic and personalized process, and every step forward is a win. In the future chapters, we'll continue to explore tasty dishes and practical ideas to boost your meal planning experience. Get ready to savor the joys of a balanced and satisfying lifestyle!

Chapter 8: Maintaining Your Weight Loss Success

Thank you for coming to this point in your journey! Achieving and maintaining weight loss success is a big deal, and in this chapter, we'll look at ways to move from active weight reduction to maintenance. We'll also discuss how to create long-term healthy lifestyle habits and why it's important to acknowledge your accomplishments as you work toward new objectives.

8.1 Transitioning from Weight Loss to Maintenance

Making some deliberate changes to your strategy and moving from the active phase of weight loss to maintenance calls for careful thought. Finding a long-term equilibrium that enables you to lead a healthy, meaningful life and maintain your ideal weight is the aim.

1. Establish Realistic Maintenance Goals: Setting attainable and long-term goals is crucial when you go into the maintenance phase. Change your attention from actively trying to lose weight to keeping your weight within a healthy, steady range. Establish objectives for sustaining your existing lifestyle, such as consistent exercise, a healthy diet, and mindful eating.

2. Monitor Your Progress: As the emphasis moves away from active weight loss, keep track of your advancement. Check in with your weight, energy, and general health on a regular basis. To keep a healthy balance, make the necessary adjustments to your behaviors if you observe any noticeable changes.

3. Adjust Caloric Intake: It could be necessary for you to modify your calorie intake once your active weight reduction has stopped. Determine how many calories you need for maintenance based on your age, exercise level, and metabolism. Try to eat just enough calories to maintain your current weight neither too many nor too few.

4. Emphasize Sustainable Habits: Give enduring behaviors that enhance your general well-being a lot of attention. Maintain a balanced and diverse diet, continue to practice mindful eating, and get frequent exercise. The basis for sustained success is laid by these behaviors.

5. Intuitive Eating: Think about making intuitive eating a part of your daily routine. Eat in reaction to physical hunger rather than other influences by paying attention to your body's signals of hunger and fullness. Intuitive eating encourages a more sustainable and natural way of eating as well as a positive relationship with food.

6. Be Flexible: Being adaptable is essential at the upkeep stage. Acknowledge that special occasions and sporadic departures from your routine are regular aspects of life. After such aberrations, be adaptable in your approach and concentrate on getting back to your healthy routine.

7. Continue Meal Prep Practices: Continue to prepare your meals as the foundation of your healthful way of living. Even while calorie restriction may not be as important, meal preparation is still a useful strategy to make sure you always have wholesome, filling meals on hand. To maintain your general well-being, keep organizing and cooking your meals ahead of time.

8.2 Long-Term Habits for a Healthy Lifestyle

The key to maintaining weight reduction success is developing enduring habits that support a happy and healthy way of life. Let's examine some essential behaviors that will promote your continued wellbeing.

1. Regular Physical Activity: Continue an enjoyable and regular exercise regimen. Frequent exercise helps people maintain their weight and is also beneficial for general health, mental health, and enhanced vigor. Selecting pursuits you enjoy will increase the likelihood that you'll persist with them over time.

2. Balanced Nutrition: Maintain your focus on a healthy diet by including a range of nutritious foods in your meals. Make sure you consume a variety of fruits, vegetables, whole grains, lean proteins, and healthy fats. To make sure you get a variety of vitamins and minerals, aim for nutrient diversity.

3. Hydration: Drink enough water throughout the day. Water is essential for several body processes, such as metabolism, digestion, and general health. Make water your main hydration source and pay attention to your needs, particularly when engaging in strenuous activity.

4. Adequate Sleep: Make it a priority to obtain enough good sleep. Sleep deprivation has an adverse effect on one's physical and mental health, which may compromise one's capacity to make wise decisions. Establish a calming bedtime ritual and strive for a regular sleep pattern.

5. Stress Management: Make use of practical stress-reduction strategies on a daily basis. Persistent stress has an effect on general health and weight control. Examine stress-relieving hobbies, yoga, deep breathing techniques, meditation, and other activities.

6. Social Support: Preserve and fortify your network of social support. Be in the company of people who support your aims or who are as committed to living a healthy lifestyle as you are. Social ties can have a good impact on your habits and help you feel like you belong.

7. Continuous Learning: By continuing your education about well-being, fitness, and nutrition, you may stay educated and involved in your journey toward better health. Stay informed about new findings, experiment with different recipes, and maintain a curiosity in methods to improve your general well-being.

8. Mindful Eating Practices: Maintain your mindful eating habits to promote a positive relationship with food. Savor the flavors of your food, pay attention to your body's signals of hunger and fullness, and develop an understanding of the emotional components of eating.

9. Set and Review Goals Regularly: Make sure you frequently assess your success and set new goals for yourself. Objectives offer guidance and inspiration. They may have to do with reaching fitness goals, experimenting with novel forms of exercise, or learning about many facets of leading a healthy lifestyle.

10. Self-Care Practices: Set aside time each day for self-care as a priority. Taking care of you, whether it's by relaxing, taking up a hobby, or engaging in joyful activities, is important for resilience and general well-being.

8.3 Celebrating Your Achievements and Setting New Goals

Rewarding yourself for your accomplishments is a crucial part of staying motivated and developing an optimistic outlook. Here's how to recognize your accomplishments and make new resolutions for ongoing development.

1. Reflect on Your Journey: Give your weight loss journey some thought. Recognize the obstacles you've surmounted, the routines you've established, and the improvements you've experienced in your life. Taking stock of your trip strengthens your resolve and fortitude.

2. Celebrate Milestones: Honor your progress and accomplishments along the road. Celebrate these accomplishments as proof of your commitment and hard work, whether it's hitting a target weight, finishing a fitness challenge, or maintaining a regular schedule of good behaviors.

3. Reward Yourself: Give yourself incentives that support your objectives. Select incentives that improve your general wellbeing rather than your appetite. This can be a weekend getaway, a spa day, or a new exercise gadget.

4. Share Your Achievements: Tell your network of supporters about your accomplishments. Sharing your achievement with others, whether it be through friends, family, or an online community, not only enables you to enjoy the compliments but also encourages and supports others as they travel through life.

5. Set New Goals: Seize the chance to establish fresh objectives for ongoing development. These objectives, which focus on various facets of your health and wellbeing, can be both short- and long-term. Establishing fresh objectives gives one direction and a sense of purpose.

6. Embrace Adaptability: Acknowledge that it's acceptable for your ambitions to change as time goes on. Accept change and be willing to modify your goals in response to shifting priorities, tastes, and situations in your life.

7. Cultivate a Positive Mindset: Maintain an optimistic outlook on the process. Pay attention to the strides you've taken, the knowledge you've gained, and the benefits to your health and wellbeing. Resilience and long-term success are facilitated by an optimistic outlook.

8. Seek Professional Guidance: Think about consulting with nutritionists, personal trainers, or health coaches for expert advice. Their knowledge may offer tailored advice, assistance, and insights as you move through the maintenance stage and establish new objectives.

9. Embody the Lifestyle: Change your mind set to one of a continuing lifestyle rather than seeing your trip as a one-time endeavor. Adopting a healthy lifestyle entails incorporating routines into your day-to-day activities in a way that seems organic and long-lasting.

10. Express Gratitude: Give thanks for the experience and the improvements in your life. Having gratitude makes you feel happy and fulfilled. Give yourself a time to acknowledge the growth and well-being you have achieved.

Recall that your path is distinct and dynamic as you embrace the maintenance stage. You'll be able to sustain your weight loss progress and advance toward total well-being by adopting these

tactics into your daily routine. We'll cover more delectable dishes

and helpful tips to improve your meal planning experience in the

next chapters. Prepare to enjoy the benefits of a happy, balanced

lifestyle for years to come!

Chapter 9: Frequently Asked Questions

This chapter will cover a number of commonly asked issues about meal planning, losing weight, and typical obstacles people may run into when trying to live a healthy lifestyle.

9.1 Common Questions about Meal Prep

1. Q: How do I start with meal prep if I've never done it before?

A: Starting with meal prep is easier than you might think. Begin by planning simple meals for the week, focusing on recipes that share common ingredients to minimize waste. Start with one or two recipes and gradually increase the variety as you become more comfortable with the process. Invest in quality food storage containers to keep your prepped meals fresh.

2. Q: Can I meal prep for the entire week, or is it better to do it more frequently?

A: While meal prepping for the entire week is possible, it may depend on the type of food you're preparing. Some ingredients and dishes stay fresh longer than others. As a general guideline, aim for a mix of fresh and freezer-friendly meals. You can do a larger meal prep session at the beginning of the week and a smaller one mid-week for added variety.

3. Q: How can I prevent my meals from becoming bland or monotonous?

A: Variety is key to preventing mealtime monotony. Explore different cuisines, flavors, and cooking techniques. Rotate your protein sources, experiment with herbs and spices, and incorporate a diverse selection of fruits and vegetables. This not only keeps your meals interesting but also ensures you receive a wide range of nutrients.

4. Q: Can I still meal prep if I have dietary restrictions or allergies?

A: Absolutely! Meal prep is highly adaptable to various dietary restrictions and allergies. Focus on recipes that align with your dietary needs, and use substitutes or modifications when necessary. There are plenty of resources and cookbooks catering to specific dietary requirements, making it easier to find recipes that suit your preferences.

5. Q: How do I prevent my vegetables from becoming soggy during meal prep?

A: To prevent vegetables from becoming soggy, consider adopting certain strategies:

Roast Instead of Steam: Roasting vegetables can help maintain their texture and flavor. Spread them out on a baking sheet and roast at a high temperature for a shorter time.

Store Separately: If possible, store sauces or dressings separately from the vegetables until you're ready to eat. This helps maintain crispness.

Opt for Sturdy Vegetables: Choose sturdy vegetables that hold up well to cooking and reheating, such as broccoli, Brussels sprouts, and bell peppers.

6. Q: How long can I store my prepped meals in the refrigerator?

A: The storage time for prepped meals in the refrigerator depends on the ingredients and their freshness. In general, most cooked meals can be stored in the refrigerator for 3-4 days. It's crucial to label containers with the preparation date and consume them within the recommended time frame to ensure freshness and safety.

7. Q: Can I freeze all types of meals, or are there exceptions?

A: While many meals can be successfully frozen, some ingredients may not fare well in the freezer. For example, foods with high water content, such as lettuce or cucumbers, tend to become mushy when thawed. Additionally, dishes with dairy-based sauces may separate upon freezing and reheating. It's best to research the freezing compatibility of specific ingredients and recipes.

8. Q: How do I avoid overcooking or undercooking my proteins during meal prep?

A: Achieving the right level of doneness in proteins requires attention to cooking times and temperatures. Invest in a kitchen thermometer to ensure proteins reach their recommended internal temperatures. Additionally, consider using a variety of cooking methods baking, grilling, and sautéing to keep things interesting and avoid monotony.

9.2 Addressing Weight Loss Concerns

1. Q: Will meal prep help me lose weight?

A: Yes, meal prep can be a powerful tool for weight loss. Planning and preparing your meals in advance give you better control over portion sizes and the nutritional content of your food. It also helps you make mindful choices and avoid impulsive, less healthy options. However, it's essential to combine meal prep with a balanced diet and regular physical activity for optimal weight loss results.

2. Q: How can I prevent overeating during meals?

A: Several strategies can help prevent overeating during meals:

Portion Control: Use smaller plates and containers to control portion sizes.

Eat Mindfully: Pay attention to your body's hunger and fullness cues. Put down your utensils between bites, chew slowly, and savor the flavors.

Stay Hydrated: Drink water throughout your meals. Sometimes, thirst can be mistaken for hunger.

Include Fiber and Protein: Meals rich in fiber and protein tend to be more satisfying, reducing the likelihood of overeating.

3. Q: Can I still enjoy my favorite foods while trying to lose weight?

A: Absolutely! Weight loss doesn't mean giving up your favorite foods entirely. It's about moderation and finding a balance that works for you. Consider incorporating your favorite foods into your meal plan occasionally, making sure they fit within your overall calorie and nutritional goals.

4. Q: I've hit a weight loss plateau. What should I do?

A: Weight loss plateaus are common and can be addressed by making adjustments to your routine:

Review Your Caloric Intake: Ensure you're in a calorie deficit.

If you've lost weight, your body may require fewer calories than when you started.

Adjust Your Exercise Routine: Modify your workout routine to include a mix of strength training and cardiovascular exercise. This can boost your metabolism and break through a plateau.

Reassess Your Meal Plan: Take a fresh look at your meal plan. Are there areas where you can improve the nutritional quality or reduce portion sizes?

Stay Consistent: Plateaus are temporary, and consistency is key. Stay committed to your healthy habits, and changes will likely follow.

5. Q: Should I follow a specific diet plan for weight loss?

A: The effectiveness of a specific diet plan depends on individual preferences, lifestyle, and health considerations. While some people find success with structured plans like keto, paleo, or intermittent fasting, others prefer a more flexible approach. The key is to choose a plan that aligns with your preferences and is sustainable in the long term.

6. Q: Is it necessary to count calories for weight loss?

A: While not everyone needs to count calories, it can be a helpful tool for creating awareness of your food intake. Tracking calories allows you to understand portion sizes and identify areas where you can make adjustments. However, it's essential to approach calorie counting with a balanced and mindful mindset to avoid developing unhealthy relationships with food.

9.3 Troubleshooting Challenges in Your Diet Plan

1. Q: I find it challenging to stick to my meal prep routine. How can I stay consistent?

A: Consistency is crucial for success in any health journey. To stay consistent with your meal prep routine:

Set Realistic Goals: Start with achievable goals and gradually build up. Setting unrealistic expectations can lead to frustration.

Create a Schedule: Plan dedicated time for meal prep in your weekly schedule, treating it as a non-negotiable appointment increases the likelihood of consistency.

Celebrate Small Wins: Acknowledge and celebrate the small victories along the way. Consistency is built through positive reinforcement.

Find Accountability: Share your goals with a friend, family member, or online community, having someone to be accountable to can boost motivation.

2. Q: I often experience cravings for unhealthy foods. How can I manage them?

A: Cravings are normal, and managing them involves a combination of strategies:

Hydrate: Drink water when cravings strike, as thirst can sometimes be mistaken for hunger.

Healthy Alternatives: Have healthier alternatives on hand to satisfy cravings. For example, if you crave sweets, opt for fruit or a small piece of dark chocolate.

Mindful Eating: Practice mindful eating by savoring each bite and paying attention to the flavors. This can help reduce impulsive eating.

Identify Triggers: Understand the triggers behind your cravings, whether they're emotional or situational. Finding alternative ways to cope with these triggers is key.

3. Q: I struggle with portion control. How can I manage this?

A: Portion control is a common challenge, but it can be addressed with mindful practices:

Use Smaller Plates: Opt for smaller plates to visually trick your mind into thinking you have a full plate.

Listen to Your Body: Pay attention to your body's hunger and fullness cues. Stop eating when you feel satisfied rather than overly full.

Pre-portion Snacks: Instead of eating directly from the package, pre-portion snacks into smaller containers to avoid mindless eating.

Include Fiber and Protein: Meals rich in fiber and protein tend to be more satisfying, making it easier to control portions.

4. Q: I struggle with meal planning and often resort to last-minute decisions. How can I improve?

A: Efficient meal planning requires some upfront effort, but it pays off in the long run:

Set a Weekly Planning Session: Dedicate a specific time each week for meal planning. This can include choosing recipes, creating a shopping list, and scheduling meal prep sessions.

Start Small: If planning for the entire week feels overwhelming, start with a few days at a time. As you become more comfortable, gradually extend your planning period.

Batch Cooking: Consider batch cooking certain components, like proteins or grains that can be used in multiple meals throughout the week. This reduces the need for extensive daily planning.

Use Planning Apps: Explore meal planning apps that provide recipes, shopping lists, and even the option to schedule your meals for the week.

5. Q: I face challenges when dining out or attending social events. How can I make healthier choices in these situations?

A: Making healthier choices in social situations involves mindful decision-making:

Preview Menus in Advance: Check restaurant menus or ask about available options before arriving. This allows you to make informed choices.

Prioritize Protein and Vegetables: Choose dishes that include lean proteins and plenty of vegetables. These options tend to be more nutrient-dense.

Control Portions: Be mindful of portion sizes, and consider sharing dishes or packing up leftovers to avoid overeating.

Stay Active: Incorporate physical activity into social events, such as taking a post-meal walk or participating in group activities.

Communicate Your Goals: Share your health and fitness goals with friends and family. Having their support can make it easier to make healthier choices.

6. Q: I'm not seeing the results I expected. What might be going wrong?

A: If you're not seeing the desired results, it's essential to assess various factors:

Caloric Intake: Review your caloric intake and ensure you're in a calorie deficit for weight loss.

Exercise Routine: Evaluate your exercise routine. Consider incorporating a mix of strength training and cardiovascular exercise to enhance results.

Sleep and Stress: Ensure you're getting sufficient sleep and effectively managing stress, as these factors can impact weight loss.

Nutritional Quality: Reassess the nutritional quality of your meals. Focus on nutrient-dense foods and a balanced diet.

Consistency: Consistency is key in any health journey. Ensure you're consistently following your meal plan and exercise routine.

Remember that progress takes time, and individual factors can influence results. If concerns persist, consulting with a healthcare professional or nutritionist for personalized guidance may be beneficial.

In summary

Preparing meals, losing weight, and pursuing a better lifestyle all require ongoing education. By answering frequently asked queries and resolving problems, your arm yourself with information and useful techniques. Keep in mind that every person's path is different, so feel free to modify these recommendations to suit your own tastes and situation. We'll look at more advice and recipes to improve your meal planning experience in the following and last chapter. Prepare to enjoy the tasty and nourishing results of a carefully planned and well-prepared meal plan!

Chapter 10: Conclusion

Thank you for finishing "The Ultimate Meal Prep Cookbook for Weight Loss: The Ultimate Beginners Guide to Eating Healthy and Achieving Your Weight Maintenance." As you come to the end of this extensive guide, think back on your experience and plan ways to maintain your healthy lifestyle after you finish the cookbook.

10.1 Reflecting on Your Journey

1. Celebrate Your Achievements: Spend some time acknowledging and appreciating the progress you've made in food planning and weight loss. Every accomplishment whether it's learning a new dish, hitting a fitness target, or reliably sticking to your diet plan is evidence of your commitment and diligence.

2. Acknowledge Challenges and Growth: Recognize the difficulties you've encountered and the knowledge you've gained thus far. Overcoming challenges is a common pathway to growth, and each one offers a chance for adaptation and learning. Accept and utilize the resilience you've acquired.

3. Consider Your Relationship with Food: Consider the changes in your relationship with food that have occurred during this journey. Have you started paying more attention to what you eat? Are the decisions you're making supporting your objectives for wellness and health? Developing a healthy connection with food and understanding it is essential for long-term wellbeing.

4. Evaluate Your Healthy Habits: Consider how well your daily routine now includes your healthy behaviors. These practices, which include meal planning, consistent exercise, and mindful eating, improve your general health. Feel proud of the improvements you've achieved and reflect on how they've shaped your way of living.

10.2 Continuing Your Healthy Lifestyle beyond the Cookbook

1. Maintain Consistency: Maintaining the gains you've made requires consistency. Continue to give your newly formed healthy habits top priority as you proceed. Maintaining consistency enables you to enjoy the long-term advantages of a healthy lifestyle in addition to reinforcing excellent behaviors.

2. Explore New Recipes and Techniques: Continue the excitement by experimenting with different meal preparation methods and dishes. There are always opportunities to find scrumptious and nutritious options in the wide world of cuisine. Savor the delight of discovering new flavors and ingredients, experimenting with cooking techniques, and venturing into world cuisines.

3. Set New Goals: Establishing fresh objectives gives your continuing journey focus and inspiration. Think about your short- and long-term objectives for your diet, exercise, and other well-being-related areas. Establishing goals helps you stay motivated and focused on ongoing personal development.

4. Stay Informed and Inspired: Keep up your knowledge on fitness, nutrition, and general health. Continue to read from reliable sources, have an open mind, and maintain your curiosity about any new advancement in the field of health and wellness. Your continuous dedication to a healthy lifestyle can be strengthened by looking for inspiration from publications, books, or even other enthusiasts.

5. Share Your Knowledge and Experience: Think about imparting your wisdom and experience to others. Your path has the power to uplift and encourage people around you, whether you share it with close friends, family, or virtual groups. Fostering a supportive and upbeat atmosphere promotes a feeling of belonging and teamwork.

6. Embrace Flexibility: Because life is dynamic, things can change. Accept adaptability in your approach to wellbeing and health. Be willing to modify your plans, schedules, and tactics in response to shifting priorities, changing life stages, or fresh revelations. You can overcome obstacles with resiliency and adaptation if you have flexibility.

7. Prioritize Self-Care: Make self-care a priority as a continuous commitment to your health. Self-care, whether it takes the form of hobbies, leisure, or joyful pursuits, is a crucial element of a healthy and satisfying lifestyle. It is equally important to look after your mental and emotional well-being as it is your physical well-being.

8. Seek Professional Guidance: If necessary, think about consulting with nutritionists, personal trainers, or health coaches for expert advice. Their knowledge can offer you individualized advice, support, and insights as you move through various stages of your health journey.

9. Cultivate Gratitude: Practice being grateful for the improvements in your life. Thank them for the healthy meals, the increased strength and vitality, and the general well-being you have developed. Having gratitude improves your experience in general and cultivates a positive outlook.

Final Thoughts

As you wrap up this comprehensive book, keep in mind that maintaining your health is an ongoing journey. A comprehensive approach to wellbeing includes the knowledge you've gained, the routines you've established, and the delectable meals you've adopted. Savor the benefits of a well-balanced and satisfying lifestyle, regardless of whether you're starting again or maintaining old routines. We appreciate you joining us on this trip, and we wish your health, happiness, and the pleasures of

delicious, wholesome meals along the way.

About the Author

Dr. Adam C. stands as a beacon of inspiration in the fields of medicine, nutrition, and self-help, with a remarkable journey that exemplifies the transformative power of healthy living. Armed with a professional master's degree in health nutrition and years of experience, Dr. C. has become a guiding light for individuals seeking to embrace vibrant well-being and lead happier lives.

From an early age, Dr. C. navigated through a myriad of health challenges that ranged from genetic predispositions to the pitfalls of unhealthy eating. His personal struggle ignited a flame of determination within him, one that was fueled by the belief that the human body possesses an incredible ability to heal and rejuvenate through the right nourishment. Through steadfast dedication, Dr. C. managed to conquer his own ailments and emerged as a living testament to the transformative potential of a well-balanced lifestyle.

What sets Dr. Adam C. apart is his rich tapestry of experiences, having been deeply immersed in groundbreaking research in health food and diet-related domains. His quest to uncover the hidden treasures of nutrients within our meals has led to groundbreaking revel actions that empower individuals to extract the maximum benefit from their dietary choices. Dr. C.'s research has not only contributed to the scientific community but has also served as a roadmap for countless individuals striving to optimize their health.

However, it is not just Dr. C.'s academic prowess that has touched lives it is his unparalleled compassion and empathy that truly make him a beacon of hope. His personal journey of triumph over adversity infuses his guidance with an authentic understanding of the challenges his readers and patients face. Dr. C. doesn't just prescribe nutritional plans; he fosters a deep connection with his audience, instilling in them the confidence to embark on their own transformative journeys.

Dr. Adam C.'s holistic approach reaches beyond the confines of traditional medicine. His insights have translated into self-help resources that empower individuals to take charge of their wellness narrative. His words resonate on paper as they do in person, making his books not mere guides, but trusted companions on the path to vitality.

In the realm of health and nutrition, Dr. C. shines as a true luminary. His core strengths lie in his ability to synthesize complex scientific findings into practical, actionable advice that individuals from all walks of life can seamlessly integrate into their routines. Dr. C.'s legacy is not just a collection of breakthroughs; it is a testament to the extraordinary potential that lies within each of us to overcome obstacles and embrace a life brimming with health, happiness, and fulfillment.

As an experienced doctor, passionate nutritionist, and empathetic author, Dr. Adam C. continues to transform lives, showing us that the journey to a healthier, happier existence is within our grasp, waiting to be unlocked through the power of informed choices and unwavering determination.